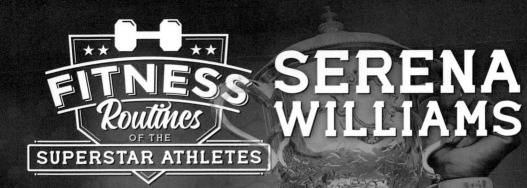

SERENA WILLIAMS

JEFF SAVAGE

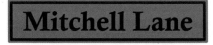

PUBLISHERS

2001 SW 31st Avenue
Hallandale, FL 33009

www.mitchelllane.com

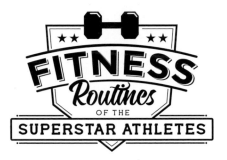

First Edition, 2020.
Author: Jeff Savage
Designer: Ed Morgan
Editor: Lisa Petrillo

Series: Fitness Routines of the Superstar Athletes
Title: Serena Williams / by Jeff Savage

Hallandale, FL : Mitchell Lane Publishers, [2020]

Library bound ISBN: 9781680204735
eBook ISBN: 9781680204742

PHOTO CREDITS: Design Elements, freepik.com, vexels.com, AP Images,

Contents

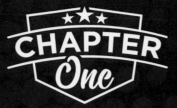

RECORD
Breaker

S erena Williams walked into the arena in Melbourne Park carrying her racket bag and a secret. She removed her headphones to hear the cheers from the crowd. Williams was about to play in the 2017 Australian Open final. She was hoping to make history. Williams was trying to win her 23rd **Grand Slam** singles title. No tennis player had won more major tournaments in the **Open Era**.

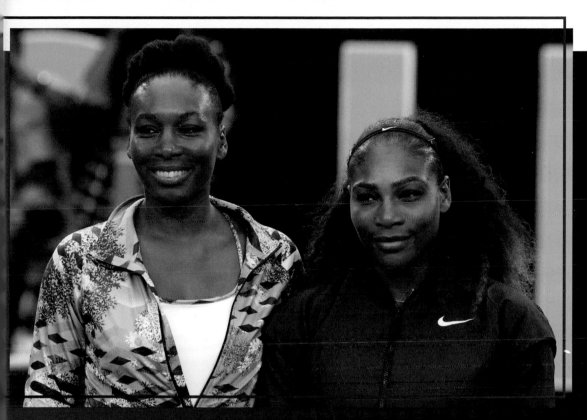

Serena Williams (*right*) and Venus before the women's singles final at the Australian Open tennis championships in January 2017.

Serena faced a familiar opponent—her sister Venus. The Williams sisters had played in tournaments against each other dozens of times. In fact, when Serena first visited Melbourne in 1998 at age 16, with braces on her teeth and braids in her hair, she lost in the second round—to Venus. The sisters knew each other's strengths and weaknesses. This match would be a challenge.

Serena and her sister traded serves and **groundstrokes**. The first set was close, with Serena winning, 6-4. The truth is, Serena expected to win. She had already won the Australian Open six times. (Venus had never won it.) Serena was playing at the top of her game. In this year's tournament, for the first time ever, Serena hadn't even lost a set. If she won this match she would be ranked No. 1 in the world—by far the oldest woman ever.

At age 35, Serena was considered an "old" player. Tennis careers are normally over by then. Steffi Graf, the player whose record Serena was hoping to break, retired at age 30. Venus is one year older than Serena, and she was still playing, but she hadn't reached a Grand Slam final in eight years. Serena had won 10 of her 22 Grand Slams after age 30. It seemed that the older she got, the *better* she got.

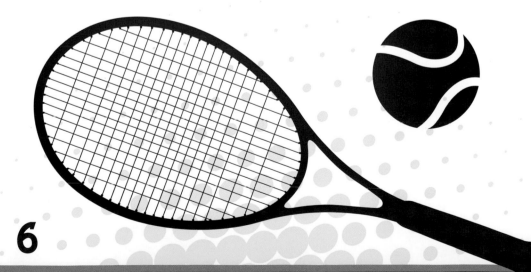

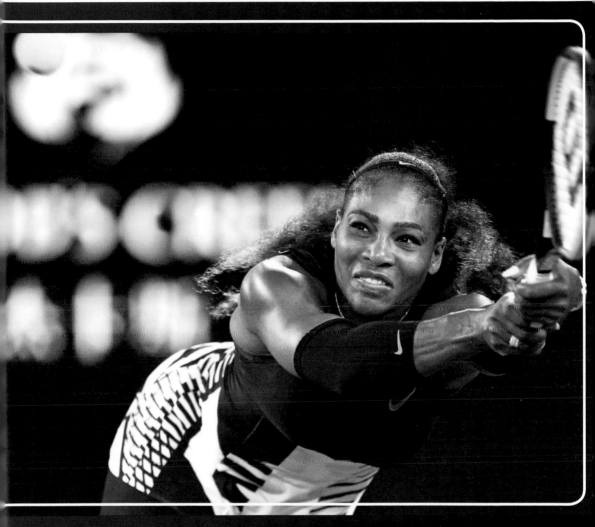

Serena Williams hits a ball against Venus Williams in the final of the Australian Open tennis tournament in Melbourne, Australia.

Serena took a 5-4 lead in the second set. She needed to win one more game to close out the match. Tied at 30-30, Serena smashed a serve that Venus barely returned. Serena ripped a two-handed backhand and Venus whacked it into the net. It was match point. Serena blasted a forehand to the baseline and Venus hit it wide. Serena had won her record-breaking title and the $3.7 million in prize money that came with it.

Tennis legends marveled at Serena's greatness at such an age. Billie Jean King tweeted: "Serena—you are a history maker and a trailblazer!" Martina Navratilova tweeted: "Unbelievable. Serena does it again. What an amazing record!" After winning the tournament, Serena revealed her secret. She was pregnant!

Fun Fact

As a young girl, Serena warmed up for practice each day by walking around the entire tennis court—on her hands (a handstand walk)!

Williams raises her trophy during the awards ceremony after her victory.

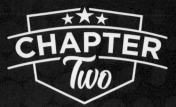

CHAPTER Two

Overcoming the ODDS

Serena Jameka Williams was born September 26, 1981, in Saginaw, Michigan. She is the youngest of five daughters born to Oracene and Richard Williams. Serena grew up with her older sisters Yetunde, Isha, Lyndrea, and Venus. The Williams family soon moved to Compton, a city with a high crime rate outside Los Angeles in Southern California. "I had to worry about all kinds of things growing up," Serena remembered. "Gangs, robberies, murders. Gun shots right outside our door. There was a lot to be afraid of. There was a lot to run away from." Richard began teaching his two youngest

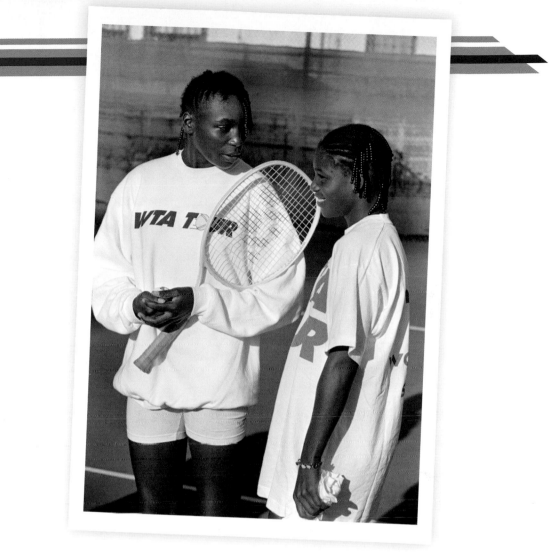

Serena Williams (*right*) and Venus as young teens in 1994 hoping to play on the WTA Tour.

daughters the game of tennis when Serena was age 3. Practices lasted two hours or longer. Both girls were home schooled to allow more time for tennis. Serena was 9 when her family moved again, this time to West Palm Beach, Florida. She entered several area tournaments and built a junior tournament record of 46-3, already making a reputation for herself.

Serena joined the Women's Tennis Association (WTA) in 1997 at age 15 and finished the season ranked 99th in the world. The following year, she reached the **quarterfinals** in six tournaments—but lost all of them. She did win two Grand Slam **mixed doubles** tournaments and teamed with her sister to win three doubles titles. Her breakout year came in 1999 when she won her first Grand Slam by defeating top-ranked Martina Hingis at the U.S. Open. She became the first African-American woman to win a major title in 41 years. Williams won the 2002 French Open, Wimbledon, and the U.S. Open, and the 2003 Australian Open to make tennis history by owning the title in all four majors at once. In 2015, she claimed her second "Serena Slam" when she won at Wimbledon to own all four major titles again.

Williams celebrates as she wins the singles match against Heather Watson of Britain, in Wimbledon, London, July 2015.

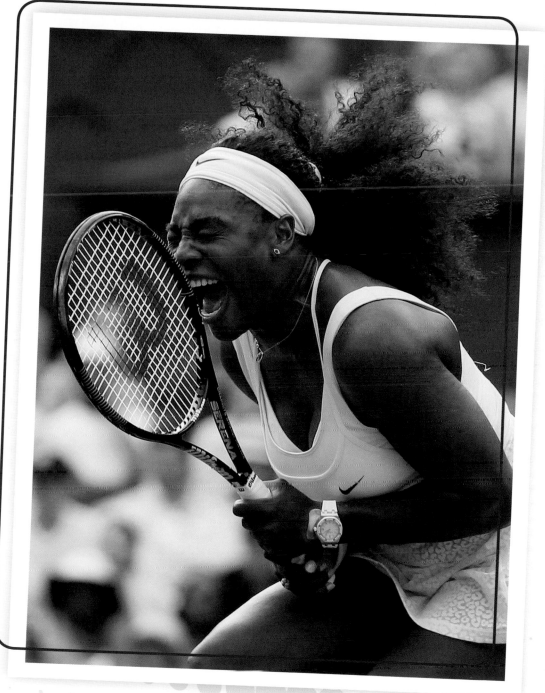

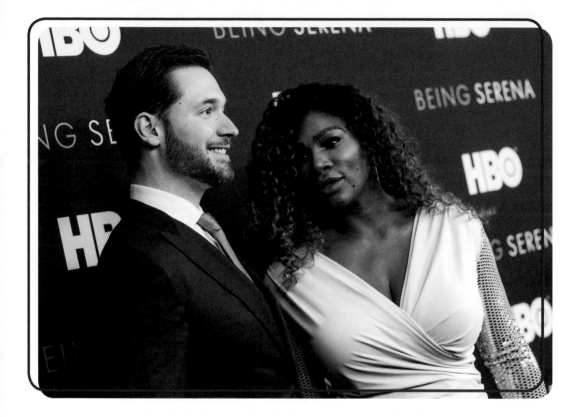

Williams and Alexis Ohanian

On September 1, 2017, Williams gave birth to daughter Alexis Olympia Ohanian Jr. (she goes by "Olympia"). She married Alexis Ohanian, a businessman who created the popular website Reddit. After giving birth, Williams suffered complications and underwent several surgeries.

Barely able to walk at first, she spent six months working her way back to health. She returned to competition at the 2018 French Open where she won her first three matches before withdrawing with a chest injury. At both Wimbledon and the U.S. Open, she roared through all her opponents all the way to the finals. Williams refused to allow illness, injury, and age to hold her back. How was this possible?

Fun Fact

Serena lived with her sister Venus for more than a decade in a mansion in Florida. In 2013, Serena bought her own mansion nearby.

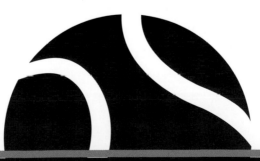

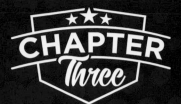

CHAPTER
Three

INTENSITY
Training

Serena Williams might be the strongest player in the history of women's tennis. She blasts groundstrokes from the baseline with such force that rallies don't last long. She converts normal returns into passing shots cross court or down the line. Her serve has been clocked at 129 miles per hour. That's the second-fastest serve of all time. Beneath her stylish outfits are rock-hard muscles. "I'm more fit than I've ever been," she told a magazine writer. "But I don't love my arms. People want more fit arms, but my arms are *too* fit. But I'm not complaining. They pay my bills."

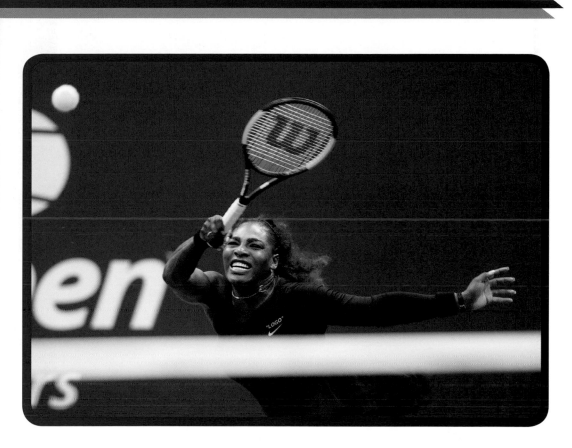

Women's Singles Finals match at the U.S.
Open in September 2018

The stress Williams puts on her body has caused injuries. She has had surgeries on her knees and feet. She has suffered other health problems, such as stomach bleeding and blood clots in her abdomen. Some of her lung tissue has been permanently destroyed. Yet as Williams approaches 40 years old, she remains at the top of her game. How?

Intensity! Williams practices and trains with a passion that matches her play in tournaments. On the court with coach Patrick Mouratoglou, she often rallies against *two* training partners. They provide a cardiovascular workout that strengthens her heart by keeping her moving from side to side and making her chase lobs and drop shots. Sometimes she tethers her wrist or body to a **resistance band**—making it harder for her to swing or move. Her two-hour practice sessions are focused on speed and endurance.

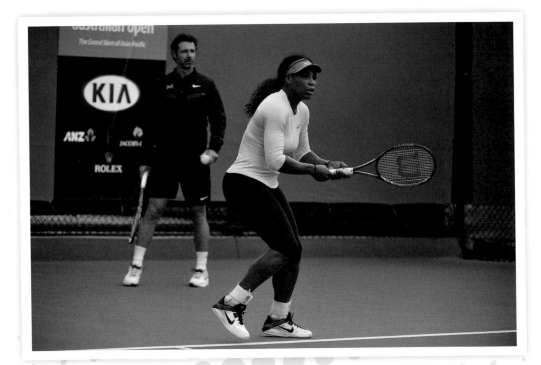

Williams trains with Patrick Mouratoglou.

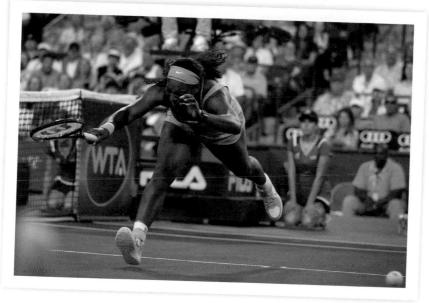

Williams dominates with her powerful lower body.

Williams makes her biggest gains in the gym. Her personal fitness trainer is Mackie Shilstone. He has trained thousands of athletes, including quarterback Peyton Manning, shortstop Derek Jeter, and other star athletes. Shilstone's workout routine for Williams targets all muscle groups. For her upper body, she does pushups, pull-downs, and dumbbell presses. She performs **plank rows** with a resistance band for three minutes without stopping. To strengthen her core (midsection), she does **rope pulls**, **bicycle crunches**, planks, and other exercises. Williams has a powerful lower body. To maintain her strength, she does barbell **squats**, dumbbell **step-ups**, dumbbell **walking lunges**, and other lifts.

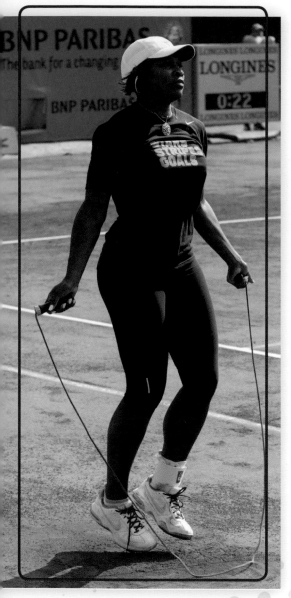

Williams skips rope while thinking about her next victory.

Williams spends much of her training time working on conditioning. In addition to practicing on the tennis court, she uses popular exercise equipment such as a stationary bike, step climber, and jump rope. But Williams admits that she does not like doing cardio work. "It's boring to me," she told a reporter. "So when I'm doing it, I think about how much I want to win. That's the only thing that keeps me going. Plus, I have to mix it up." Tennis players use one side of their body more than the other. To correct that imbalance, Williams practices a discipline called **Pilates**. She takes **Zumba** dance classes. She even runs up hills and swings her tennis racket in a swimming pool.

Williams doesn't win every match. When she loses, she works out even harder. After she lost a match in California in 2018, for instance, she went to a nearby court the next day to hit 300 serves. "With a defeat, when you lose, you get up, you try again, you make it better," she explained. "I've always said a champion isn't about how much they win, but it's about how they recover from their downs, whether it's an injury or whether it's a loss."

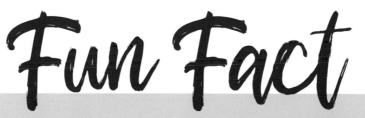

Fun Fact

Serena speaks four languages (French, Spanish, Italian, and of course, English.) After French Open matches she often gives her interviews in French.

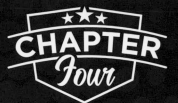

CHAPTER Four

Healthy LIVING

W illiams has a large frame. She stands 5 feet 9 inches tall, and weighs 160 pounds. A simple formula using height and weight indicates she is overweight. But that is not the case. Williams is muscular. She has little body fat. Muscle weighs more than fat. Williams carries "extra" weight due to her sturdy physique. She has been teased for it, but she knows what matters. "We're taught that we have to look a certain way," Williams explained. "We're told what's beautiful and what's not, and that's not right. Since I don't look like every other girl, it took me a while to be okay with that. I love who I am now, but it definitely wasn't easy."

Williams is careful with what she eats. She consumes a healthy combination of protein and carbohydrates. For protein she eats grilled or baked chicken and fish, eggs, milk, and other dairy products. For carbohydrates she enjoys potatoes, rice, fruits, and vegetables. Her typical day might look like this:

Breakfast—a toasted Ezekiel bread sandwich with almond butter, and fruit such as strawberries or a tangerine.

Lunch—a salad with lettuce and spinach leaves, mandarin oranges, cherry tomatoes, onions, pita croutons, and sliced almonds.

Dinner—a grilled chicken breast, brown rice, steamed vegetables, and green tea.

Williams also eats healthy snacks in between regular meals. She usually eats six times a day to keep her body humming. During tournament weeks, she eats plenty of nuts, beans, lentils, and sprouted quinoa. Before a match she might consume a green smoothie with protein powder and vegetables like kale. But while she eats mainly nutritious foods, she does occasionally enjoy "comfort foods" such as shrimp and grits with butter, fried chicken, and banana pudding. "I try to eat healthy all the time," she told a reporter, "but I can never turn down a good piece of cherry pie."

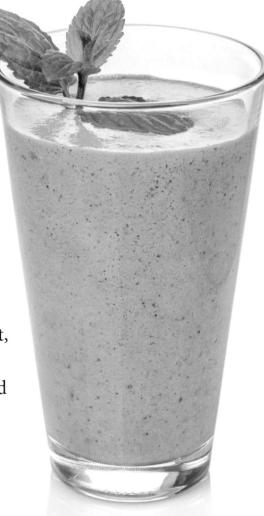

Williams says she is allergic to wheat. She tries to eat a gluten-free diet. Gluten is a mix of proteins found in wheat, barley, oats, and other grains. She doesn't like to use the word "diet," but instead prefers the term "lifestyle change."

Maintaining a healthy body is important to Williams, and so is having a healthy mind. To achieve this, she practices **Bikram yoga**. The movements and positions are good for blood flow and flexibility, but she enjoys it for the calming effect it has on her mind. She also likes to write. She has nine million followers on Instagram and millions more on Twitter. But it is a different form of writing that eases her mind. She likes to write her personal thoughts in a journal that only she reads. "Writing down your feelings in a notebook or journal can help clear out negative thoughts and emotions that keep you feeling stuck," she explained.

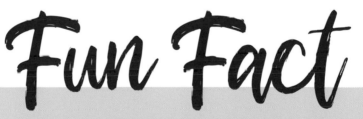

Serena is part owner of the Miami Dolphins. In 2009, she and her sister Venus became the first African-American women to own part of a National Football League (NFL) team.

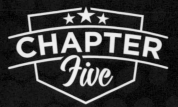

CHAPTER Five

BUILT for Success

Serena Williams has been famous for nearly two decades. In 2002, a national magazine listed her as one of the world's "Most Intriguing People." In 2015, she was named another magazine's "Sportsperson of the Year"—the first female athlete to be so honored in 32 years. That same year, a poll named her the fourth greatest athlete in history—behind Michael Jordan, Babe Ruth, and Muhammad Ali. She has appeared in more than a dozen television shows and even has her own television series.

Williams has won nearly $90 million in prize money—more than twice that of any other player in history. She earns millions more each year in **endorsements** by sponsoring companies that sell technology, furniture, music equipment, sporting goods, and cars. She even has her own clothing line. She donates a lot of her money. The Serena Williams Foundation builds schools around the world and provides **scholarships** for underprivileged students in the United States. Williams gives speeches each year to support an end to homelessness, poverty, and domestic abuse. On and off the tennis court, she works hard at everything she does.

"People see me on the court only as a superhero, grunting and winning," she told a reporter. "But I am not a robot. I have a heart and I bleed. I work hard. My story isn't over. For me, there's always another mountain to climb. There's something really cool about setting a goal and meeting it. You have to work hard for success. Everything comes at a cost. Just what are you willing to pay for it?"

Fun Fact

Serena put her 2017 Australian Open trophy on a shelf in Olympia's bedroom since her daughter was "with her" when she won the title.

AWARDS

U.S. Open Champion
6 times (1999, 2002, 2008, 2012, 2013, 2014)

French Open Champion
3 times (2002, 2013, 2015)

Wimbledon Champion
7 times (2002, 2003, 2009, 2010, 2012, 2015, 2016)

Australian Open Champion
7 times (2003, 2005, 2007, 2009, 2010, 2015, 2017)

Sportswoman of the Year (Laureus)
4 times (2003, 2010, 2016, 2018)

Sportsperson of the Year (*Sports Illustrated*)
(2015)

Olympic Champion
4 times (singles: 2012; doubles: 2000, 2008, 2012)

TIMELINE

1981 — born in Saginaw, Michigan

1997 — started competing on the WTA Tour

1999 — won first U.S. Open title (first Grand Slam title)

2000 — won first Olympic gold medal doubles title

2002 — won first French Open title

2002 — won first Wimbledon title

2003 — won first Australian Open title

2012 — won gold medal at London Olympics

2014 — won sixth French Open title

2015 — won third French Open title

2016 — won sixth Wimbledon title

2017 — won seventh Australian Open title

GLOSSARY

bicycle crunches Exercise in which you are flat on your back with your legs in the air and you move them as if pedaling a bike

Bikram yoga Exercise program, performed in a heated room, in which you put your body in 26 specific positions designed to increase blood flow

endorsement Money paid by a company to someone in exchange for promoting its product

Grand Slam One of four major tournaments held each year (Australian Open, French Open, Wimbledon, U.S. Open)

groundstroke Shot hit after it bounces with a forehand or backhand stroke

mixed doubles Match between one male and one female on each side

Open Era The current period in tennis beginning in 1968 when professionals were allowed to compete in major tournaments and prize money was awarded

Pilates Series of movements performed in a certain order to strengthen the core and improve balance

plank rows Exercise in which you hold steady in a pushup position with one hand while pulling a resistance band toward you with the other

quarterfinals Stage of a tournament in which four matches remain

resistance band Rope made of rubber or latex that stretches like a thick rubber band, some with a handle at both ends

rope pulls Exercise in which you grip a thick rope with both hands and pull it toward you

scholarship Money and other aid given to students to help pay to attend school

squats Exercise performed from a standing position in which you lower your body, as though sitting in a chair, and then stand back up

step-ups Exercise in which you step onto a platform about knee-height, step back down, and repeat a number of times

walking lunges Exercise in which you step forward and lower your body and then stand back up, often while holding dumbbells

Zumba Dance workout done to music in which class members follow an instructor's moves

FURTHER READING

Byrant, Howard. *Sisters & Champions: The True Story of Venus and Serena Williams.* New York: Philomel Books, 2018.

Fishman, Jon. *Serena Williams.* Minneapolis: Lerner Publications, 2016.

Nelson, Kristen Rajczak. *Serena Williams: Tennis Star.* New York: Enslow Publishers, 2017.

Shepherd, Jodie. *Serena Williams: A Champion on and off the Court.* New York: Children's Press, 2017.

ON THE INTERNET

www.SerenaWilliams.com
Williams's official site

www.usta.com
The United States Tennis Association's official site

www.wtatennis.com
The Women's Tennis Association's official site

INDEX

ABOUT the AUTHOR

Jeff Savage is the award-winning author of more than 200 books for young readers. A former sportswriter for the San Diego Union-Tribune, Jeff's books have been read by millions. Jeff lives with his wife, Nancy, sons Taylor and Bailey, and dogs Tunes, Coach, Ace, Champ, Tank, and Lexi (that's six!) in Folsom, California. Jeff met Serena Williams in 1999 and has been following her career ever since.